Healing Herbs of the Zodiac

Tony White / Samuel H. Weir

HIPPYDIPPY
GURU

www.hippydippyguru.com

ISBN: 978-1-7343858-4-7

DEDICATION

To all those individuals who have their feet firmly set on the ground ~ but, at the same time, with their eyes fixed always to the stars!

CONTENTS

ACKNOWLEDGMENTS

I with to thank the miraculous work and teachings of the late, great herbalist/astrologer **Samuel H. Weir**, without whom this book could never have been made possible. ~ *Tony White*

1 ASTROLOGY

Astrology is not *'science'* as we know it in this day and age - but neither is it *'superstition'* either. (At least not at its highest level of expression.) Serious astrological thinkers draw from a knowledge of centuries of study and observed provings, bringing about a body of knowledge and understanding concerning each individual born in a certain place, on a certain day and at a certain time. In that way, no two astrological Birth Charts are the same and each involves a great deal of probing and individual discovery. Consequently, the very highest practitioners of the art take a lifetime to practice it with confidence. So doing they ultimately learn to recognize it primarily as a unique vehicle of inner understanding that can help in a healing or counseling process - one which may give greater clarity as to an individual's unfolding life journey. The true use of the art of astrology is therefore far, far removed from that of the popular media's *'Sun Signs'* or other commercial/cult panderings.

... .

Most people know their own *'Sun Sign'* from the popular media but very few know what this really means to their way of self knowledge and life being. Neither do they know that to get a full picture of a person other factors, such as *'Moon Sign'*, *'Rising Sign'* and the position of all the other *'Planets'* in the *'Zodiac'* and *'Astrological Houses'*, need to be considered also. History is filled with great thinkers and innovators with an astrological perspective - from *Johannes Kepler* to Isaac Newton - while a number of more contemporary scientists, therapists, philosophers and physicians use astrology secretly in their work, choosing to avoid the uninformed public attacks that mentioning the fact would bring about. Artists, poets, musicians and creative individuals of all kinds have, in the main, had less reticence in expressing their inspiration. Historically however, many brave individuals have been pilloried, persecuted and even killed for their belief in the art of astrology, even though quite often their belief has equally embraced the highest spiritual, ethical or moral motives.

2 NICHOLAS CULPEPER

One of the greatest *(and yet most vilified by the establishment in his time)* practitioners of healing astrology was the 17th-century botanist and medical herbalist, **Nicholas Culpeper**. Culpeper – a Christian Puritan throughout his life - believed that there was an inextricable, almost divine, connection between the ever-changing order of the heavens and the healing gifts of God's earth. Challenging the monarchy, privileged society and even the entire medical establishment throughout his short lifetime, he chose to cure *(often 'miraculously' in the eyes of many)* the poor. He preferred to educate them on taking responsibility for their own health, rather than bankrupting themselves by paying impossibly huge fees to the invariably ineffective physicians of their time. *'Culpeper's Complete Herbal and English Physician'* is a book he published during his lifetime which is packed with botanical and astrological information that best reflects a summation of his life's work. So effective and valued is its wisdom, that it is still in print today! Culpeper has also been called the *'Father of Midwifery'* in that he was committed to safe childbirth in an age when such things were not so. He published *'A Directory for Midwifes: or a Guide for Women in Their Conception, Bearing and Suckling of Children'*, many of the basic tenants from which are still respected today. It is not surprising that his knowledge of birth and knowledge of lives beyond birth through astrology went hand in hand.

3 HEALING HERBS OF THE ZODIAC

The late, great Samuel H. Weir was the nearest thing to Nicholas Culpeper in the latter part of the 20th-century. He often achieving outstanding results with his most challenging patients - often those the medical authorities had given up on - through his great knowledge of herbs and astrology. Although Weir lived in virtual poverty himself, he would never charge for his services, seek fame or publicity and dispensed his prescribed herbs for a price that was less than they could be bought anywhere else. His enduring belief was that "God has given me this gift, and the people who most need me have nowhere else to go, so how can I charge to make them well?"

Anthony Richardson was a successful artist who's own mother had been miraculously cured by Samuel H. Weir at a time when there was no hope of recovery in any other way. So impressive was the transformation that his mother displayed that Richardson asked the aged herbalist to teach him the basics of astrology and herbs, which was exactly what occurred for some time. At one point Richardson asked his mentor to suggest 12 healing herbs he believed most closely defined in nature the 12 Signs of the Zodiac. So inspired was the artist by the response that he conceived 12 pen & ink illustrations that best reflected this knowledge.

Richardson's completed series was published as a limited edition set of greetings cards & prints that were successful at the time – and in their own small way they helped support the East London herbal practice for a while longer. Sadly, this was the only series that Richardson produced during Samuel H. Weir's lifetime, after which the artwork collected dust on his studio shelf for some considerable amount of time. ....

Now 40 years later, the *'Healing Herbs of the Zodiac'* designs have been rediscovered and released again through this book form – as well as through a series of beautiful *cards*, *prints* other *selective products* via Dandelion Arts. By owning these herb designs it is believed that many individuals will once again be able to enjoy the beauty and the wisdom they contain. Ultimately it is hoped that every owner of the 12 *'Healing Herbs of the Zodiac'* designs will find the same special inspiration in their lives that Anthony Richardson found in his all those years before.

4 ARIES

Born between March 20th ~ April 19th.

(Note: If your birthday is close to either of these two dates we recommend you consult an astrological ephemeris for the year of your birth to find an accurate 'Sun Sign' placement.)

Rosemary - Rosmarinus officinalis. *ruled by the sign of Aries.* ♈

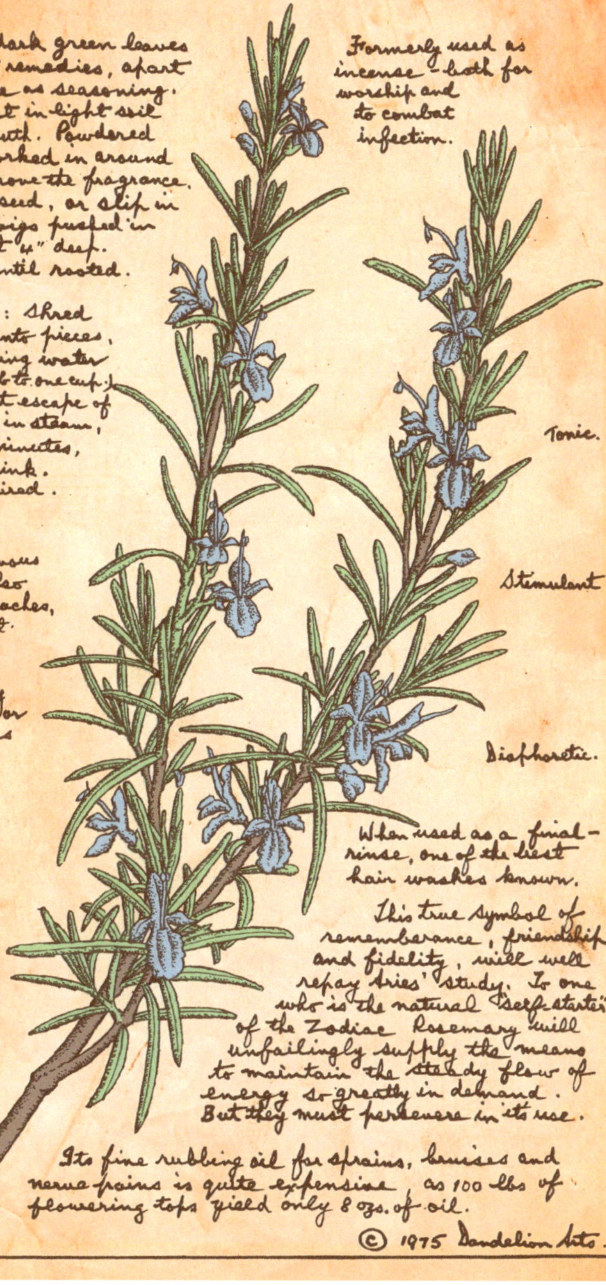

Rosemary's dark green leaves are excellent remedies, apart from their use as seasoning. It grows best in light soil and facing South. Powdered eggshells worked in around the roots improve the fragrance. Grows from seed, or slip in August. 6" twigs pushed in to earth about 4" deep. Keep moist until rooted.

Rosemary Tea: Shred fresh leaves into pieces, pour on boiling water (3 teaspoons herb to one cup.) Cover to prevent escape of volatile oil, in steam, infuse for 10 minutes, strain and drink. Repeat as required.

Special uses: To relieve nervous depression also nervous headaches, as well as that type of colic preceeding or following any anticipated or actual nervous stress.

Formerly used as incense - both for worship and to combat infection.

Tonic.

Stimulant

Diaphoretic.

When used as a final-rinse, one of the best hair washes known.

This true symbol of rememberance, friendship and fidelity, will well repay Aries' study. To one who is the natural 'self-starter' of the Zodiac Rosemary will unfailingly supply the means to maintain the steady flow of energy so greatly in demand. But they must persevere in its use.

Its fine rubbing oil for sprains, bruises and nerve pains is quite expensive, as 100 lbs of flowering tops yield only 8 ozs. of oil.

Note: No one person is 100% representative of their Zodiac Sign. Most people will know their personal 'Sun Sign' – i.e. The part of the Zodiac the sun is in at their moment of birth. However, fewer people realize that the 'Moon Sign' and 'Rising Sign' (the Sign of the Zodiac that is located over the eastern horizon at their moment of birth) - plus the Zodiac locations of Mercury, Venus, Mars, etc. - can have a huge impact on a person's way of being too.... ... ...

Those with a strong Aries drive in their astrological ***birth chart*** tend to be concerned with initiating *new activities*. The instinct is to *lead*, *pioneer* or *be first* in any venture they undertake. The pure Aries spirit knows *no fear*, has *little caution* and instinctively seeks to *rush in* (where angels fear to tread?) in any situation that attracts their attention. Challenges that tend to arise in their lives can often be a result of their inherent *restlessness* or *impulsiveness*. According to the ancient astrologers, the part of the body that Aries has greatest association with is the *head*. This can often be witnessed in Aries types through anything from them constantly *banging their heads* as a child, or *headaches* in adulthood through extreme *mental activity*.

As part of this 'Rosemary' herb card indicates... *"The medicinal herb Rosemary is perfect for the extreme Aries spirit in that it has the power to 'relieve nervous depression, also nervous headaches, as well as that type of colic preceding or following an anticipated or actual nervous stress."*.... .....

5 TAURUS

Born between ***April 19th ~ May 20th.***

(Note: If your birthday is close to either of these two dates we recommend you consult an astrological ephemeris for the year of your birth to find an accurate 'Sun Sign' placement.)

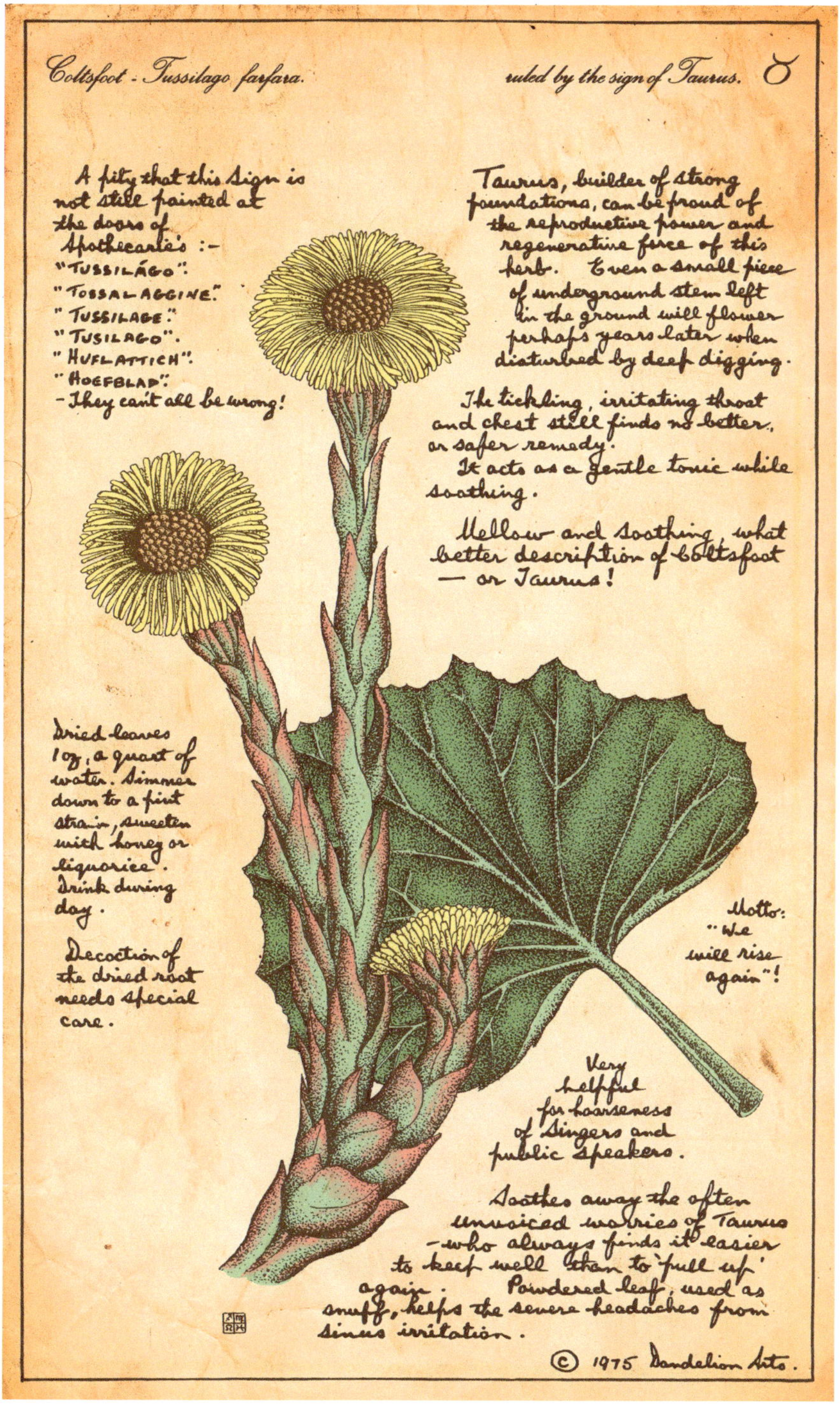
Coltsfoot - Tussilago farfara.
ruled by the sign of Taurus. ♉
A pity that this Sign is not still painted at the doors of Apothecarie's :- "TUSSILÁGO". "TOSSALAGGINE." "TUSSILAGE." "TUSILAGO". "HUFLATTICH". "HOEFBLAD". - They can't all be wrong!
Taurus, builder of strong foundations, can be proud of the reproductive power and regenerative force of this herb. Even a small piece of underground stem left in the ground will flower perhaps years later when disturbed by deep digging.
The tickling, irritating throat and chest still finds no better, or safer remedy. It acts as a gentle tonic while soothing.
Mellow and soothing, what better description of Coltsfoot — or Taurus!
Dried leaves 1oz, a quart of water. Simmer down to a pint strain, sweeten with honey or liquorice. Drink during day.
Decoction of the dried root needs special care.
Motto: "We will rise again"!
Very helpful for hoarseness of Singers and public speakers.
Soothes away the often unvoiced worries of Taurus - who always finds it easier to keep well than to 'pull up' again. Powdered leaf, used as snuff, helps the severe headaches from sinus irritation.
© 1975 Dandelion Arts.

Note: No one person is 100% representative of their Zodiac Sign. Most people will know their personal 'Sun Sign' – i.e. The part of the Zodiac the sun is in at their moment of birth. However, fewer people realize that the 'Moon Sign' and 'Rising Sign' (the Sign of the Zodiac that is located over the eastern horizon at their moment of birth) - plus the Zodiac locations of Mercury, Venus, Mars, etc. - can have a huge impact on a person's way of being too. .

That said, someone with a strong Taurus influence tends to be the most *down to earth* of all the signs. Although often quite *stubborn*, the Taurus type is nevertheless invariably extremely *reliable*, *steadfast* and *loyal*. The Taurus way is to *rarely lose their temper* and be *patient* with things and people. However, if pushed too far that placid Taurus nature can suddenly turn *angry* and even *explosive*. The Taurus type is more than happy to undertake any *practical task* that involves *long and prolonged hard work*. However, they can also be a lover of all *creature comforts*, so may *not be the fastest* at completing what they have set their mind to do. The core motivation of a Taurus being is to *build* for future *security needs*. The ruling planet of Taurus is Venus. …

…

As part of this 'Coltsfoot' herb card indicates... "*Taurus, builder of strong foundations, can be proud of the reproductive power and regenerative force of this herb. Even a small piece of underground stem left in the ground will flower perhaps years later when disturbed by deep digging.*"… ....

6 GEMINI

Born between ***May 22nd ~ June 21st.***

(Note: If your birthday is close to either of these two dates we recommend you consult an astrological ephemeris for the year of your birth to find an accurate 'Sun Sign' placement.)

Wall Germander - Teucrium chamaedrys. *ruled by the sign of Gemini.* II

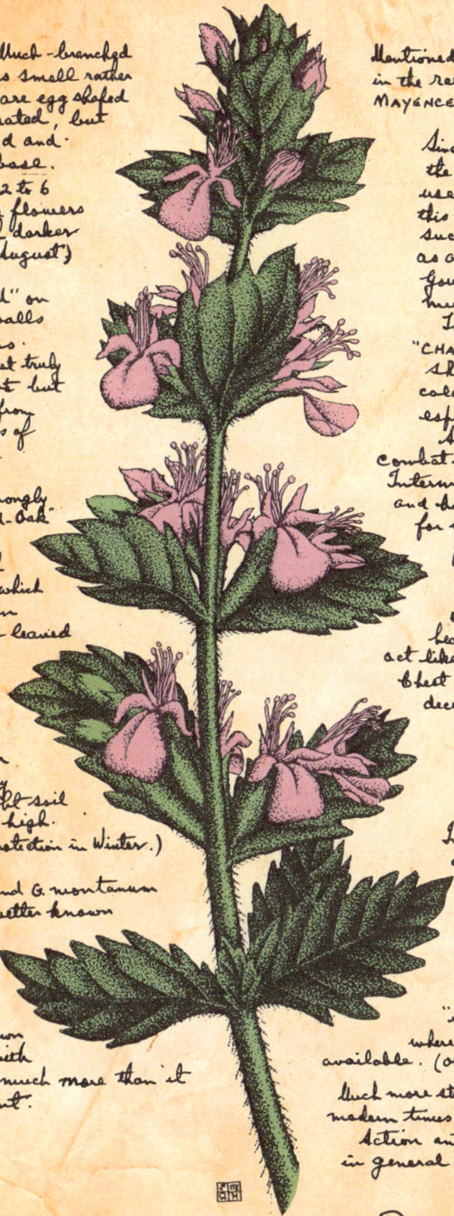

Perennial. Much-branched stem. Leaves small rather like Garlic, are egg shaped cut and serrated, but wedge-shaped and entire at base.

Whorls of 2 to 6 large purple flowers marked with darker lines (July/August)

Found "wild" on pillars and walls of old ruins.

Probably not truly a wild plant but an escapee from earliest days of cultivation.

Sometimes wrongly called "Ground-Oak"

Do not confuse with Wood-Sage which has also been called Sage-leaved Germander.

A very pleasant and very useful Rock-garden plant, easily grown on light soil and 9" to 12" high. (Needs some protection in Winter.)

(G. polium and G. montanum are perhaps better known but not so useful.)

Could be grown and used with advantage much more than it is at present.

Mentioned as "GAMANDRÉE" in the rare old Herbal of MAYENCE. (1485.)

Since Emperor Charles the Fifth's successful use of decoction of this herb (for 60 successive days) as a specific for his Gout, it has been much so used.

The French name "CHASSEE-FIEVRE" shows its value in cold or damp areas especially.

Also useful to combat weakness in Intermittent Fevers and has been used often for skin disorders following on debilitated states.

Excellent for continual nervous headaches, and will act like Horehound, for Chest soreness if the decoction be sweetened with honey and taken Hot.

Slightly aperient.

In general an activator, helping to maintain the activity of the "tribe" of Gemini.

Is even of "Airborne" growth where little soil is available. (old walls, etc.)

Much more study needed in modern times.

Action anti-inflammatory in general.

***Note: No one person is 100% representative of their** Zodiac Sign. Most people will know their personal 'Sun Sign' – i.e. the part of the Zodiac the Sun is in at their moment of birth. However, fewer people realize that the 'Moon Sign' and 'Rising Sign' (the Sign of the Zodiac that is located over the eastern horizon at their moment of birth) - plus the Zodiac locations of Mercury, Venus, Mars, etc. - can have a huge impact on a person's way of being too....   ...*

That said, someone with a strong Gemini influence in their birth chart has the facility of being a *strong communicator*. The Gemini spirit loves nothing more than to *talk*, to *learn* and to *read* about many things. Known as the *Jack-of-all-trades* (but master of none?) the qualities of *reason*, *logic*, *facts* & *figures* are 'food' for the Gemini driven individual. Often *clever* and *witty*, Gemini types will often make-up for their *lack of emotional warmth* by their *bright and breezy* approach to life…… ……….

As part of this 'Wall Germander' herb card indicates... *"Excellent for continual nervous headaches and will act like 'Horehound' for chest soreness if the decoction be sweetened with honey and taken hot."*

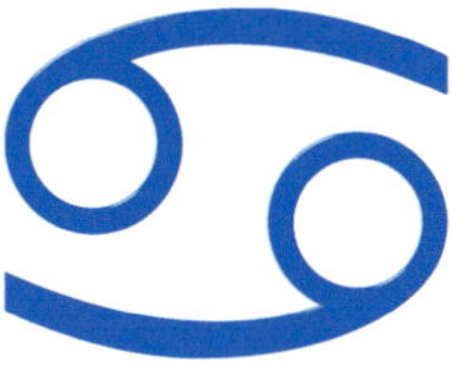

7 CANCER

Born between ***June 20th ~ July 22nd.***

(Note: If your birthday is close to either of these two dates we recommend you consult an astrological ephemeris for the year of your birth to find an accurate 'Sun Sign' placement.)

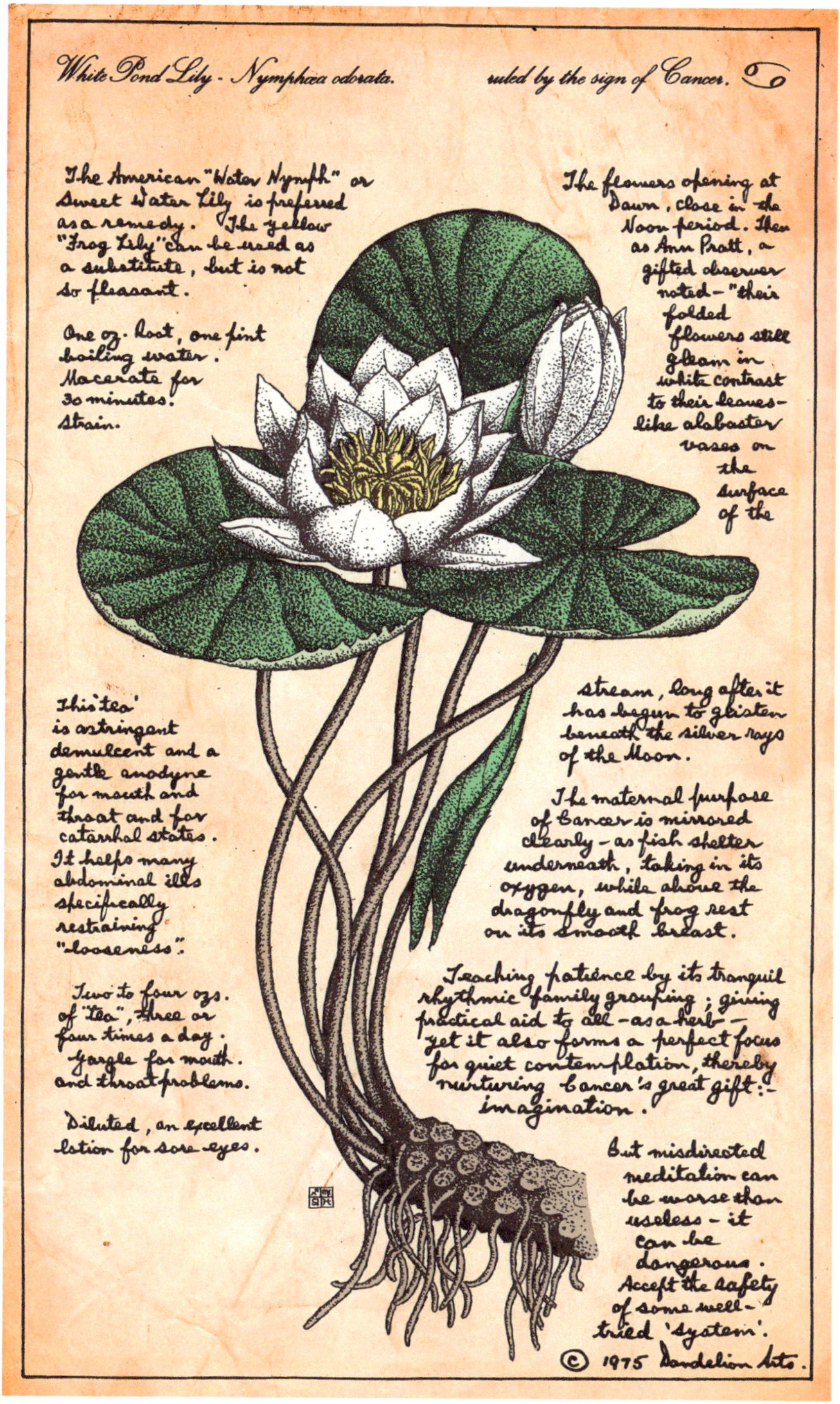
White Pond Lily - Nymphœa odorata.
ruled by the sign of Cancer. ♋
The American "Water Nymph" or Sweet Water Lily is preferred as a remedy. The yellow "Frog Lily" can be used as a substitute, but is not so pleasant.
One oz. Root, one pint boiling water. Macerate for 30 minutes. Strain.
The flowers opening at Dawn, close in the Noon period. Then as Ann Pratt, a gifted observer noted - "their folded flowers still gleam in white contrast to their leaves - like alabaster vases on the surface of the stream, long after it has begun to glisten beneath the silver rays of the Moon.
This 'tea' is astringent demulcent and a gentle anodyne for mouth and throat and for catarrhal states. It helps many abdominal ills specifically restraining "looseness".
Two to four ozs. of "tea", three or four times a day. Gargle for mouth and throat problems.
Diluted, an excellent lotion for sore eyes.
The maternal purpose of Cancer is mirrored clearly - as fish shelter underneath, taking in its oxygen, while above the dragonfly and frog rest on its smooth breast.
Teaching patience by its tranquil rhythmic family grouping; giving practical aid to all - as a herb - yet it also forms a perfect focus for quiet contemplation, thereby nurturing Cancer's great gift:- imagination.
But misdirected meditation can be worse than useless - it can be dangerous. Accept the safety of some well-tried 'system'.
© 1975 Dandelion Arts.

Note: No one person is 100% representative of their *Zodiac Sign. Most people will know their personal 'Sun Sign' – i.e. the part of the Zodiac the Sun is in at their moment of birth. However, fewer people realize that the 'Moon Sign' and 'Rising Sign' (the Sign of the Zodiac that is located over the eastern horizon at their moment of birth) - plus the Zodiac locations of Mercury, Venus, Mars, etc. - can have a huge impact on a person's way of being too....* ...

That said, those with a strong Cancerian personality are the naturally *maternal*, with a deep impulse to *feed* and *nurture* others. This kind of impulse is *sensitive to changing moods* and *environments* around them and will often *protect* their sensitivity to a threatening world by creating a *hard shell of apparent toughness* around themselves. *Intuitive* and often *psychic*, Cancerian types are acutely aware of their need for *self protection* and will as a consequence significantly immerse themselves in *home matters*, working on the principle that a Cancerian's home is their castle!.... .

As part of this 'White Pond Lily' herb card indicates... "*The maternal purpose of Cancer is mirrored clearly - as fish shelter underneath, taking in its oxygen, while above the dragonfly and frog rest on its smooth breast.*"

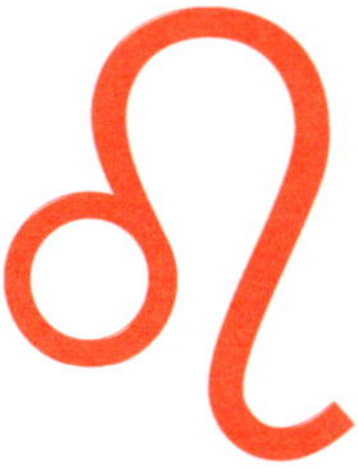

8 LEO

Born between ***July 22nd ~ August 22nd.***

(Note: If your birthday is close to either of these two dates we recommend you consult an astrological ephemeris for the year of your birth to find an accurate 'Sun Sign' placement.)

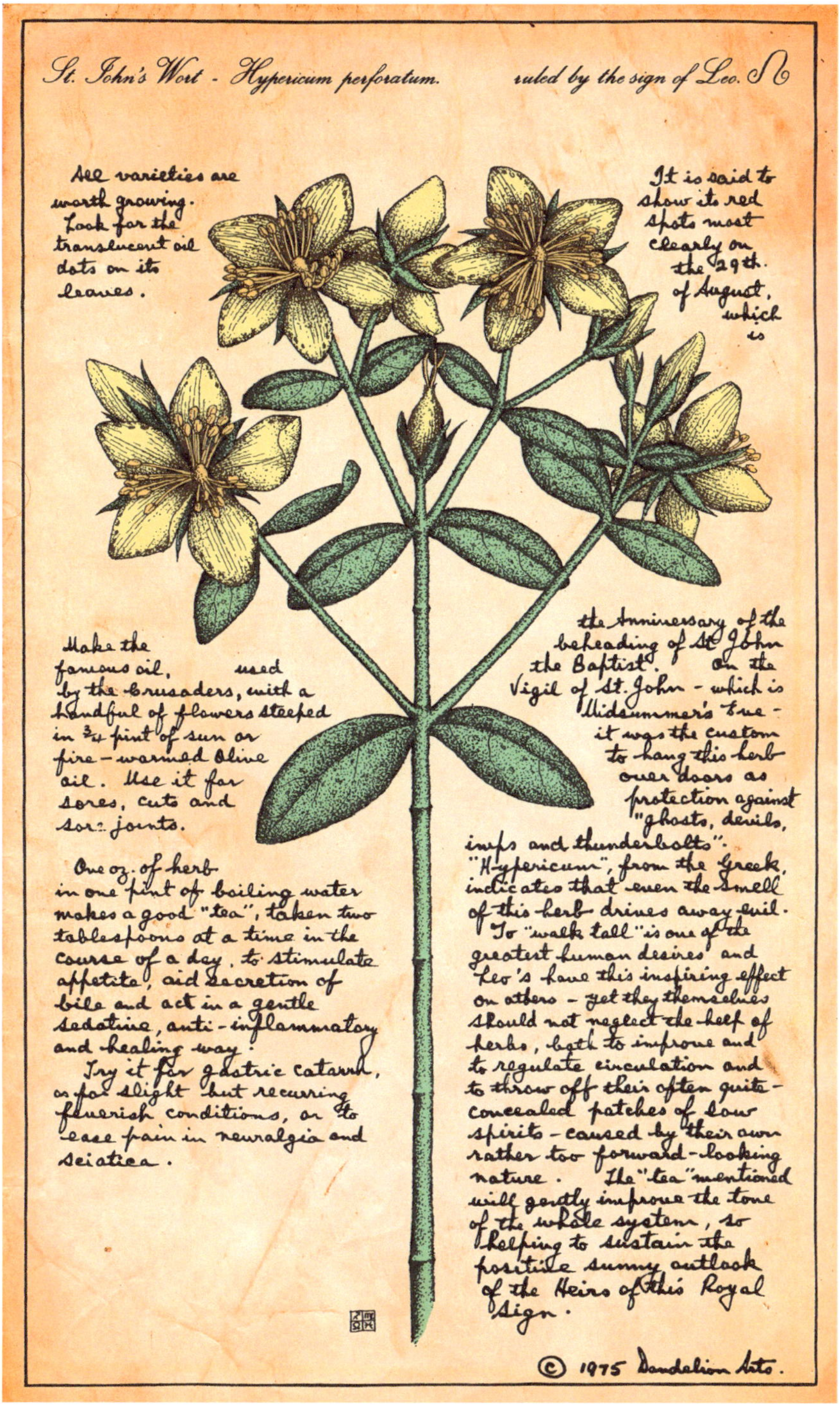
St. John's Wort - Hypericum perforatum. ruled by the sign of Leo. ♌
All varieties are worth growing. Look for the translucent oil dots on its leaves.
It is said to show its red spots most clearly on the 29th. of August, which is the Anniversary of the beheading of St John the Baptist. On the Vigil of St. John - which is Midsummer's Eve - it was the custom to hang this herb over doors as protection against "ghosts, devils, imps and thunderbolts". "Hypericum", from the Greek, indicates that even the smell of this herb drives away evil. To "walk tall" is one of the greatest human desires and Leo's have this inspiring effect on others - yet they themselves should not neglect the help of herbs, both to improve and to regulate circulation and to throw off their often quite-concealed patches of low spirits - caused by their own rather too forward-looking nature. The "tea" mentioned will gently improve the tone of the whole system, so helping to sustain the positive sunny outlook of the Heirs of this Royal Sign.
Make the famous oil, used by the Crusaders, with a handful of flowers steeped in ¾ pint of sun or fire-warmed Olive oil. Use it for sores, cuts and sore joints.
One oz. of herb in one pint of boiling water makes a good "tea", taken two tablespoons at a time in the course of a day, to stimulate appetite, aid secretion of bile and act in a gentle sedative, anti-inflammatory and healing way. Try it for gastric catarrh, or for slight but recurring feverish conditions, or to ease pain in neuralgia and sciatica.
© 1975 Dandelion Arts.

***Note: No one person is 100% representative of their** Zodiac Sign. Most people will know their personal 'Sun Sign' – i.e. the part of the Zodiac the Sun is in at their moment of birth. However, fewer people realize that the 'Moon Sign' and 'Rising Sign' (the Sign of the Zodiac that is located over the eastern horizon at their moment of birth) - plus the Zodiac locations of Mercury, Venus, Mars, etc. - can have a huge impact on a person's way of being too.... ...*

That said, someone of a Leo disposition, first and foremost, *needs to be noticed.* These spirited types are never willingly *ignored in a crowd* and take a great deal of *pride* in themselves and their opinions. They have often be described as the most *theatrical* or *attention-seeking* members of the Zodiac family. Leo types love to *rule* and can be hurt if they do not gain the *recognition* that they feel they deserve. *Loyal* and *warm* in their affections, Leo driven types are *born leaders,* with often the *strength of will* or *warmth* to inspire others too....... ..

As part of this 'St. John's Wort' herb card indicates... *"To 'walk tall' is one of the greatest human desires and Leo's have this inspiring effect on others. Yet they themselves should not neglect the help of herbs, both to improve and to regulate circulation and throw off their often quite concealed patches of low spirits - caused by their own rather too forward-looking nature."*

♍

9 VIRGO

Born between ***August 22nd ~ September 22nd.***

(Note: If your birthday is close to either of these two dates we recommend you consult an astrological ephemeris for the year of your birth to find an accurate 'Sun Sign' placement.)

Eyebright - Euphrasia officinalis. *ruled by the sign of Virgo.* ♍

There is a steady demand for this miniature herb (2 in. to 1 ft. high). Collect in flowers and dry so as to preserve colour of flower and leaves.

It can compete well even with the roots of grass, from which it is said to draw strength.

Its use both as a lotion and as a "tea" has long been proved of value. It is known to act as a gentle safe astringent and will reduce many kinds of inflammation.

'Tea' made - one oz. to one pint boiling water, and taken in wine-glassful doses in the day will lessen catarrh any-where in the system.

The "tea" can also be used for compresses and, when cool, as an eye-lotion. For the latter the liquid should be strained through very fine material.

It often proves a specific remedy for simple conjunctivitis.

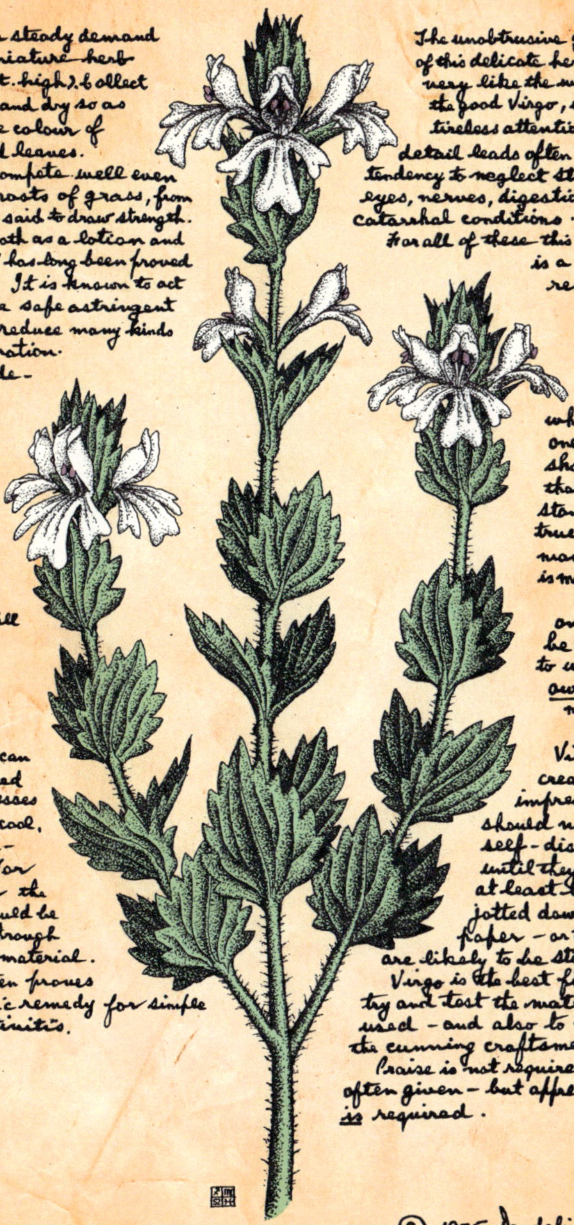

The unobtrusive growth of this delicate herb is very like the work of the good Virgo, whose tireless attention to detail leads often to a tendency to neglect strain of eyes, nerves, digestion and catarrhal conditions.

For all of these this herb is a good remedy.

In any group it is Virgo who is the one who should see that the standard of true craft-manship is maintained. They ask only to be allowed to use their <u>own</u> methods.

Virgo's creative impressions should not be self-dissected until they have at least been jotted down on paper - or they are likely to be still-born.

Virgo is the best fitted to try and test the materials used - and also to provide the cunning craftsmen.

Praise is not required - nor often given - but appreciation <u>is</u> required.

***Note: No one person is 100% representative of their** Zodiac Sign. Most people will know their personal 'Sun Sign' – i.e. the part of the Zodiac the Sun is in at their moment of birth. However, fewer people realize that the 'Moon Sign' and 'Rising Sign' (the Sign of the Zodiac that is located over the eastern horizon at their moment of birth) - plus the Zodiac locations of Mercury, Venus, Mars, etc. - can have a huge impact on a person's way of being too.... ...*

That said, a typical Virgo type is one who Is *humble* and often *self-effacing.* If Leo is born to rule, then *Virgo* is *born to serve.* If Leo has to be 'number one' then Virgo is more content to be *'number two'* – or the 'power behind the throne. Humble Virgo types delight in nothing more than to being *helpful* and *efficient* in their *service* to others. They often have a fine *attention to detail,* which can easily turn into a *nit-picking fussiness* or *worry* if their search for perfection is frustrated, unexpressed or unappreciated. Above all else, the Virgo spirit loves to *analyze* and can be naturally drawn to all forms of *health* and *work* issues. ...
......

As part of this 'Eyebright' herb card indicates... *"The unobtrusive growth of this delicate herb is very like the work of the good Virgo, who's tireless attention to detail leads often to a tendency to neglect strain of the eyes, nerves, digestion and catarrhal conditions. For all of these this herb is a good remedy."*

10 LIBRA

Born between ***September 22nd ~ October 23rd.***

(Note: If your birthday is close to either of these two dates we recommend you consult an astrological ephemeris for the year of your birth to find an accurate 'Sun Sign' placement.)

Wall Pennywort - Cotyledon umbilicous. *ruled by the sign of Libra.* ♎

This beautiful little herb grows well in dry positions in the rock garden. It seems to have been somewhat neglected by Herbalists in England during the past seventy years or so but is still in use, in some States in America, as a balancing factor when using say Horsetail Rush with other Diuretics to alleviate symptoms of kidney and bladder ailments.

They use the name 'Kidneywort' which we apply to a different herb.

One ounce of herb to one pint of boiling water makes a useful 'tea'.

Just simmer a little if using externally as a lotion for pimples or inflamed skin.

A cupful or two of the 'tea' is sufficient for an adult's daily dose.

Divide the plant in Spring or Autumn

or grow from seed - in heat - in the Spring.

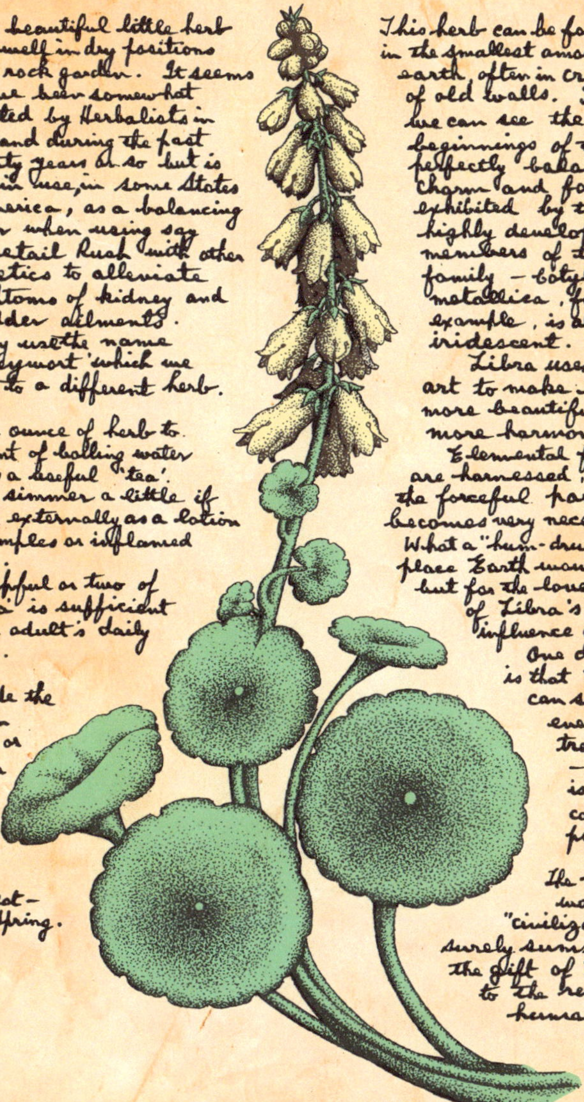

This herb can be found in the smallest amount of earth, often in crannies of old walls. In this we can see the clear beginnings of the perfectly balanced charm and form exhibited by the highly developed members of this family - Cotyledon metallica, for example, is almost iridescent.

Libra uses every art to make life more beautiful and more harmonious.

Elemental forces are harnessed, so that the forceful partner becomes very necessary.

What a "hum-drum" place Earth would be but for the loveliness of Libra's influence on it.

One danger is that Libra can sometimes even excuse treachery - if it is only carried out politely!

The very word "civilization" surely sums up the gift of Libra to the rest of humanity.

Note: No one person is 100% representative of their Zodiac Sign. Most people will know their personal 'Sun Sign' – i.e. The part of the Zodiac the sun is in at their moment of birth. However, fewer people realize that the 'Moon Sign' and 'Rising Sign' (the sign of the Zodiac that is located over the eastern horizon at their moment of birth) - plus the Zodiac locations of Mercury, Venus, Mars, etc. - can have a huge impact on a person's way of being too.. …

That said, those driven with a strong Libran influence tend to posses an inherent *sense of balance* and *social justice.* Libran types love to *weigh-up* all the opposing issues and are therefore often uncomfortable if asked to 'go out on a limb' or make a *committed decision. Harmony* is the paramount need of the Libran spirit, hence their often strong instincts of employing *diplomacy* and *tact* whenever possible. The Libran type also loves *beauty*, but can often be *lazy* when it comes to everyday chores.… ……..

As part of this 'Wall Pennywort' herb card indicates... *"Libra uses every art to make life more beautiful and more harmonious. Elemental forces are harnessed, so that the forceful partner becomes very necessary. What a 'hum-drum' place Earth would be but for the loveliness of Libra's influence on it."*

♏

11 SCORPIO

Born between ***October 23rd ~ November 21st.***

(Note: If your birthday is close to either of these two dates we recommend you consult an astrological ephemeris for the year of your birth to find an accurate 'Sun Sign' placement.)

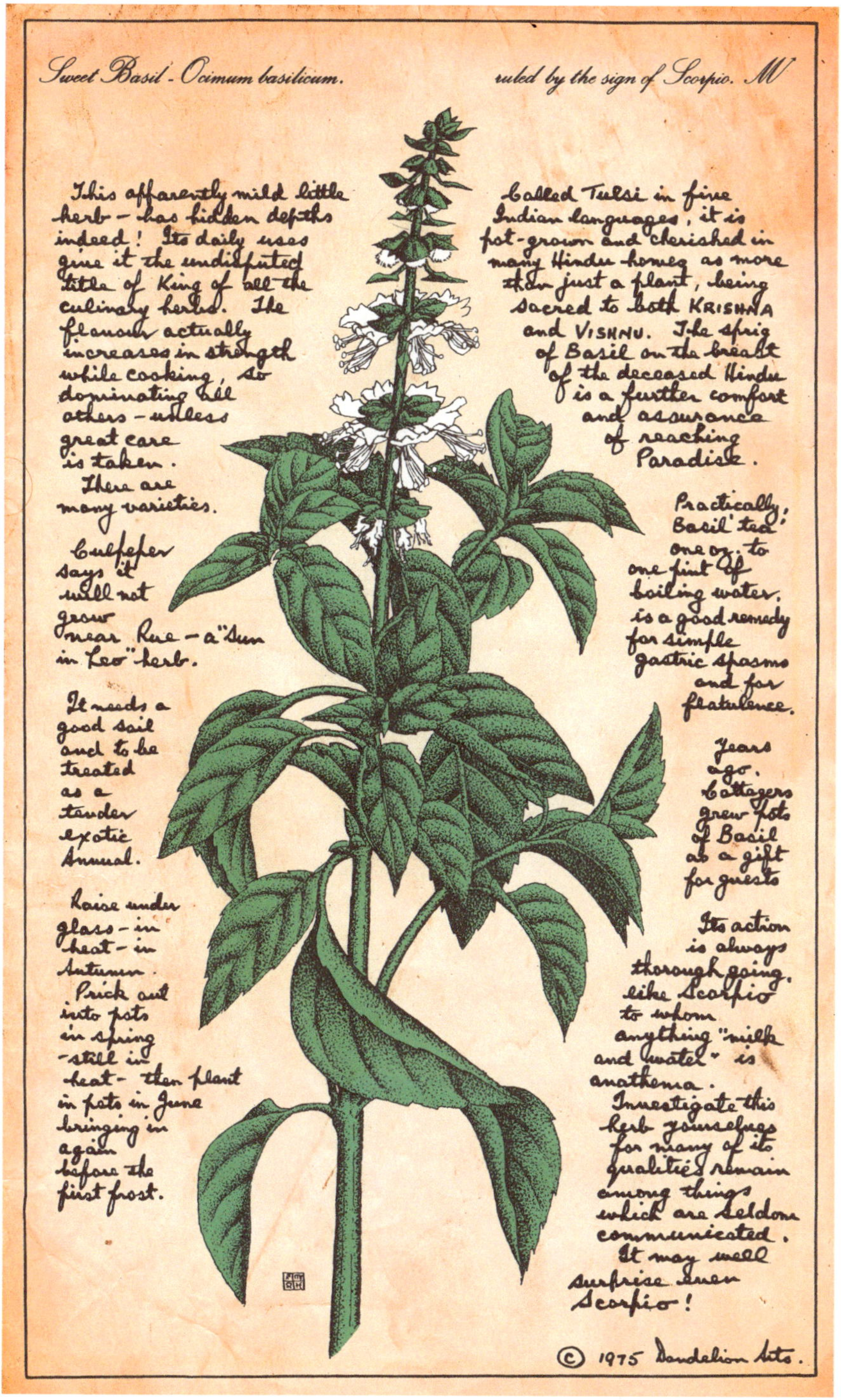
Sweet Basil - Ocimum basilicum.
ruled by the sign of Scorpio. ♏
This apparently mild little herb - has hidden depths indeed! Its daily uses give it the undisputed title of King of all the culinary herbs. The flavour actually increases in strength while cooking, so dominating all others - unless great care is taken.
There are many varieties.
Culpeper says it will not grow near Rue - a "Sun in Leo" herb.
It needs a good soil and to be treated as a tender exotic Annual.
Raise under glass - in heat - in Autumn.
Prick out into pots in spring - still in heat - then plant in pots in June bringing in again before the first frost.
Called Tulsi in five Indian languages, it is pot-grown and cherished in many Hindu homes as more than just a plant, being sacred to both KRISHNA and VISHNU. The sprig of Basil on the breast of the deceased Hindu is a further comfort and assurance of reaching Paradise.
Practically; Basil tea: one oz. to one pint of boiling water, is a good remedy for simple gastric spasms and for flatulence.
Years ago, Cottagers grew pots of Basil as a gift for guests
Its action is always thorough going, like Scorpio to whom anything "milk and water" is anathema.
Investigate this herb yourselves for many of its qualities remain among things which are seldom communicated.
It may well surprise even Scorpio!
© 1975 Dandelion Arts.

Note: No one person is 100% representative of their Zodiac Sign. Most people will know their personal 'Sun Sign' – i.e. The part of the Zodiac the sun is in at their moment of birth. However, fewer people realize that the 'Moon Sign' and 'Rising Sign' (the sign of the Zodiac that is located over the eastern horizon at their moment of birth) - plus the zodiac locations of Mercury, Venus, Mars, etc. - can have a huge impact on a person's way of being too.... ...

That said, the Scorpio natural instinct is to be *dark*, *probing* and *intense*. A Scorpio type can be *deeply perceptive* and are often motivated by a *compulsive need to control* their own *powerful emotions*. They have a passion for exploring anything that is *hidden* or *concealed* including their own *deep emotions & feelings*. At the lower end of the spectrum, Scorpio types can be prone to *jealosy* and often find it difficult to deal with their own darker emotions. Heroic and enduring, Scorpio types will of *brood in silence* when they are hurt or in pain. *death* and *sex* have an additional fascination for the Scorpio temperament, which they express in various degrees of intensity. ......

As part of this 'Sweet Basil' herb card indicates... *"Its action is always thorough going, like Scorpio to whom anything 'milk and water' is anathema. Investigate this herb yourself for many of its qualities remain among things which are seldom communicated. It may well surprise even Scorpio!"*

12 SAGITTARIUS

Born between ***November 21st ~ December 21st.***

(Note: If your birthday is close to either of these two dates we recommend you consult an astrological ephemeris for the year of your birth to find an accurate 'Sun Sign' placement.)…

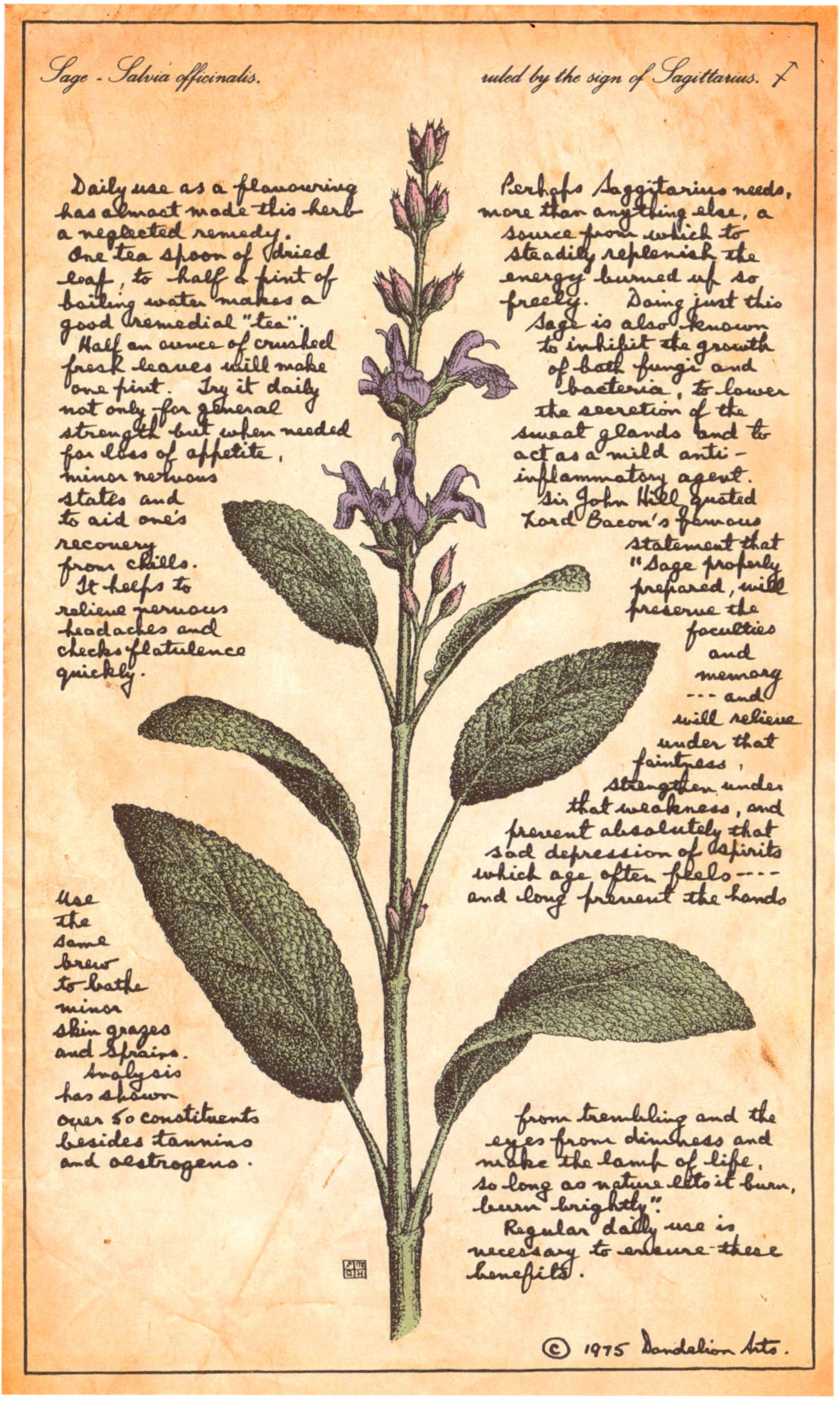
Sage - Salvia officinalis.
ruled by the sign of Sagittarius. ♐
Daily use as a flavouring has almost made this herb a neglected remedy.
One tea spoon of dried leaf, to half a pint of boiling water makes a good remedial "tea".
Half an ounce of crushed fresh leaves will make one pint. Try it daily not only for general strength but when needed for loss of appetite, minor nervous states and to aid one's recovery from chills.
It helps to relieve nervous headaches and checks flatulence quickly.
Use the same brew to bathe minor skin grazes and sprains.
Analysis has shown over 50 constituents besides tannins and oestrogens.
Perhaps Saggitarius needs, more than anything else, a source from which to steadily replenish the energy burned up so freely. Doing just this Sage is also known to inhibit the growth of both fungi and bacteria, to lower the secretion of the sweat glands and to act as a mild anti-inflammatory agent.
Sir John Hill quoted Lord Bacon's famous statement that "Sage properly prepared, will preserve the faculties and memory --- and will relieve under that faintness, strengthen under that weakness, and prevent absolutely that sad depression of spirits which age often feels --- and long prevent the hands from trembling and the eyes from dimness and make the lamp of life, so long as nature lets it burn, burn brightly".
Regular daily use is necessary to ensure these benefits.
© 1975 Dandelion Arts.

Note: No one person is 100% representative of their Zodiac sign. Most people will know their personal 'Sun Sign' – i.e. The part of the Zodiac the sun is in at their moment of birth. However, fewer people realize that the 'Moon Sign' and 'Rising Sign' (the Sign of the Zodiac that is located over the eastern horizon at their moment of birth) - plus the Zodiac locations of Mercury, Venus, Mars, etc. - can have a huge impact on a person's way of being too.... ...

That said, the Sagittarius native is a *freedom* and *don't tie me down* one. Sagittarian types have an inherent and restless search for *understanding, truth* and *faith*. They love to *travel* too (both in mind and body) and delight a great deal in any kind of *adventure of discovery*. There is invariably a smile on the face of the Sagittarian individual, often ensuring that they are the most likeable of Signs. However, if this free living spirit is not contained or wisely directed there can be significant *dissipation of energies* too.... ….. …..

As part of this 'Sage' herb card indicates... *"Perhaps Sagittarius needs, more than anything else, a source from which to steadily replenish the energy burned up so freely. Doing just this Sage is also known to inhibit the growth of both fungi and bacteria, to lower the secretion of the sweat glands and to act as a mild anti-inflammatory agent."*.

♑

13 CAPRICORN

Born between ***December 21st ~ January 19th.***

(Note: If your birthday is close to either of these two dates we recommend you consult an astrological ephemeris for the year of your birth to find an accurate 'Sun Sign' placement.)

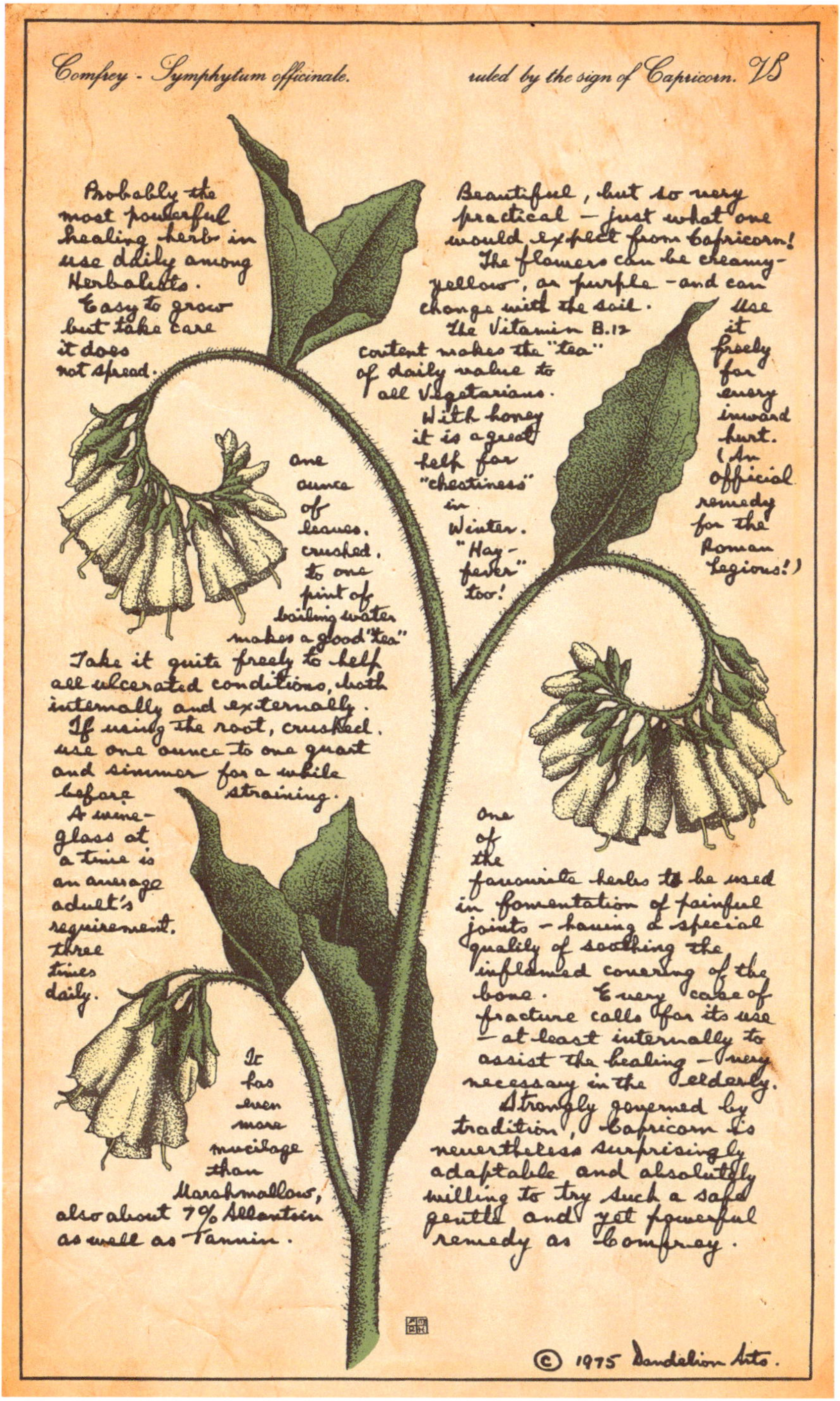
Comfrey - Symphytum officinale.
ruled by the sign of Capricorn. ♑
Probably the most powerful healing herb in use daily among Herbalists.
Easy to grow but take care it does not spread.
Beautiful, but so very practical – just what one would expect from Capricorn!
The flowers can be creamy-yellow, or purple – and can change with the soil.
The Vitamin B.12 content makes the "tea" of daily value to all Vegetarians.
With honey it is a great help for "chestiness" in Winter. "Hay-fever" too!
Use it freely for every inward hurt. (An Official remedy for the Roman Legions!)
one ounce of leaves, crushed, to one pint of boiling water makes a good "tea"
Take it quite freely to help all ulcerated conditions, both internally and externally.
If using the root, crushed, use one ounce to one quart and simmer for a while before straining.
A wine-glass at a time is an average adult's requirement, three times daily.
One of the favourite herbs to be used in fomentation of painful joints – having a special quality of soothing the inflamed covering of the bone. Every case of fracture calls for its use – at least internally to assist the healing – very necessary in the elderly.
Strongly governed by tradition, Capricorn is nevertheless surprisingly adaptable and absolutely willing to try such a safe gentle and yet powerful remedy as Comfrey.
It has even more mucilage than Marshmallow, also about 7% Allantoin as well as Tannin.
© 1975 Dandelion Arts.

Note: No one person is 100% representative of their Zodiac sign. Most people will know their personal 'Sun Sign' – i.e. The part of the Zodiac the sun is in at their moment of birth. However, fewer people realize that the 'Moon Sign' and 'Rising Sign' (the Sign of the Zodiac that is located over the eastern horizon at their moment of birth) - plus the Zodiac locations of Mercury, Venus, Mars, etc. - can have a huge impact on a person's way of being too.... ... .

A classic Capricorn individual is concerned with *law*, *order* and *maintaining the status quo*. This is the most *conservative* and *ambitious* of all the Zodiac signs, believing that *hard work* and a *patient determination* to get them where their *ambition* takes them. Their *cautious* and *prudent* nature can sometimes give way to a *cold* and *mean* disposition if blocked or unfulfilled. At the same time, there is a *profound need to preserve* the *forces of justice* with the Capricornian type with the *letter of the law* needing to be *respected.* ... .

As part of this 'Comfrey' herb card indicates... "*strongly governed by tradition, Capricorn is nevertheless surprisingly adaptable and absolutely willing to try such a safe, gentle and yet powerful remedy as Comfrey.*"...... .....

14 AQUARIUS

Born between ***January 19th ~ February 18th.***

(Note: If your birthday is close to either of these two dates we recommend you consult an astrological ephemeris for the year of your birth to find an accurate 'Sun Sign' placement.)

Valerian - Valeriana officinalis. *ruled by the sign of Aquarius.* ♒

Give it a rich loamy soil kept moist by mulching. Protect against cats - they love to roll in it!

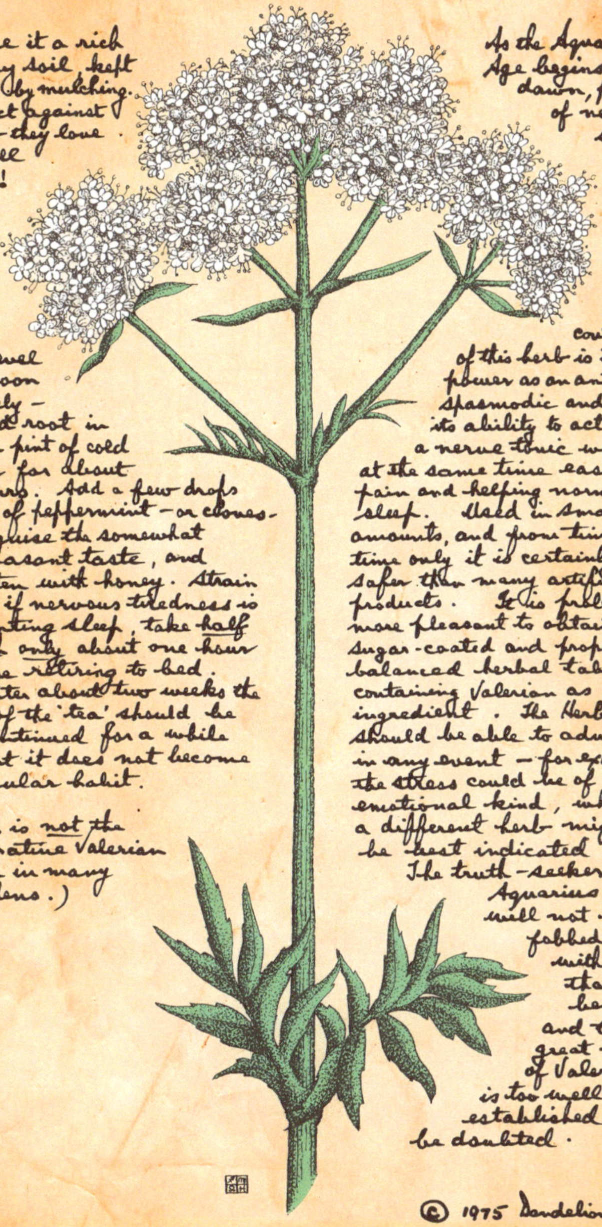

As the Aquarian Age begins to dawn, problems of nerve-stress appear more than ever before.

The great contribution of this herb is its power as an anti-spasmodic and in its ability to act as a nerve tonic while at the same time easing pain and helping normal sleep. Used in small amounts, and from time to time only it is certainly much safer than many artificial products. It is probably more pleasant to obtain sugar-coated and properly balanced herbal tablets containing Valerian as one ingredient. The Herbalist should be able to advise you in any event - for example the stress could be of an emotional kind, where a different herb might be best indicated.

The truth-seeker, Aquarius, will not be fobbed off with less than the best - and the great value of Valerian is too well established to be doubted.

To make "tea" soak one level teaspoon of finely-chopped root in half a pint of cold water for about 18 hours. Add a few drops of oil of peppermint - or cloves - to disguise the somewhat unpleasant taste, and sweeten with honey. Strain and, if nervous tiredness is preventing sleep, take <u>half a cup only</u> about one hour before retiring to bed.

After about two weeks the use of the 'tea' should be discontinued for a while so that it does not become a regular habit.

(This is <u>not</u> the decorative Valerian found in many gardens.)

Note: No one person is 100% representative of their Zodiac sign. Most people will know their personal 'Sun Sign' – i.e. The part of the Zodiac the sun is in at their moment of birth. However, fewer people realize that the 'Moon Sign' and 'Rising Sign' (the Sign of the Zodiac that is located over the eastern horizon at their moment of birth) - plus the Zodiac locations of Mercury, Venus, Mars, etc. - can have a huge impact on a person's way of being too.... .....

That said, Aquarius individuals are *idealistic* and *progressive* in their thinking. With their *independence of spirit* there is a strong need for *individual freedom* and *personal expression.* Yet this can be coupled with a marked *sympathy for the rights of others* – especially animals. Sometimes and Aquarian native's solutions to problems are *not always practical* or *sound.* Nevertheless, the Aquarian impulse is to be the *true scientist* of the zodiac, where an *unbiased pursuit of truth* is absolutely paramount.... ...

As part of this 'Valerian' herb card indicates... *"as the 'Aquarian age' begins to dawn, problems of nerve-stress appear more than before. The great contribution of this herb is its power as an anti-spasmodic and in its ability to act as a nerve tonic while at the same time easing pain and helping normal sleep."*

♓

15 PISCES

Born between ***February 18th ~ March 20th*****.**

(Note: If your birthday is close to either of these two dates we recommend you consult an astrological ephemeris for the year of your birth to find an accurate 'Sun Sign' placement.)

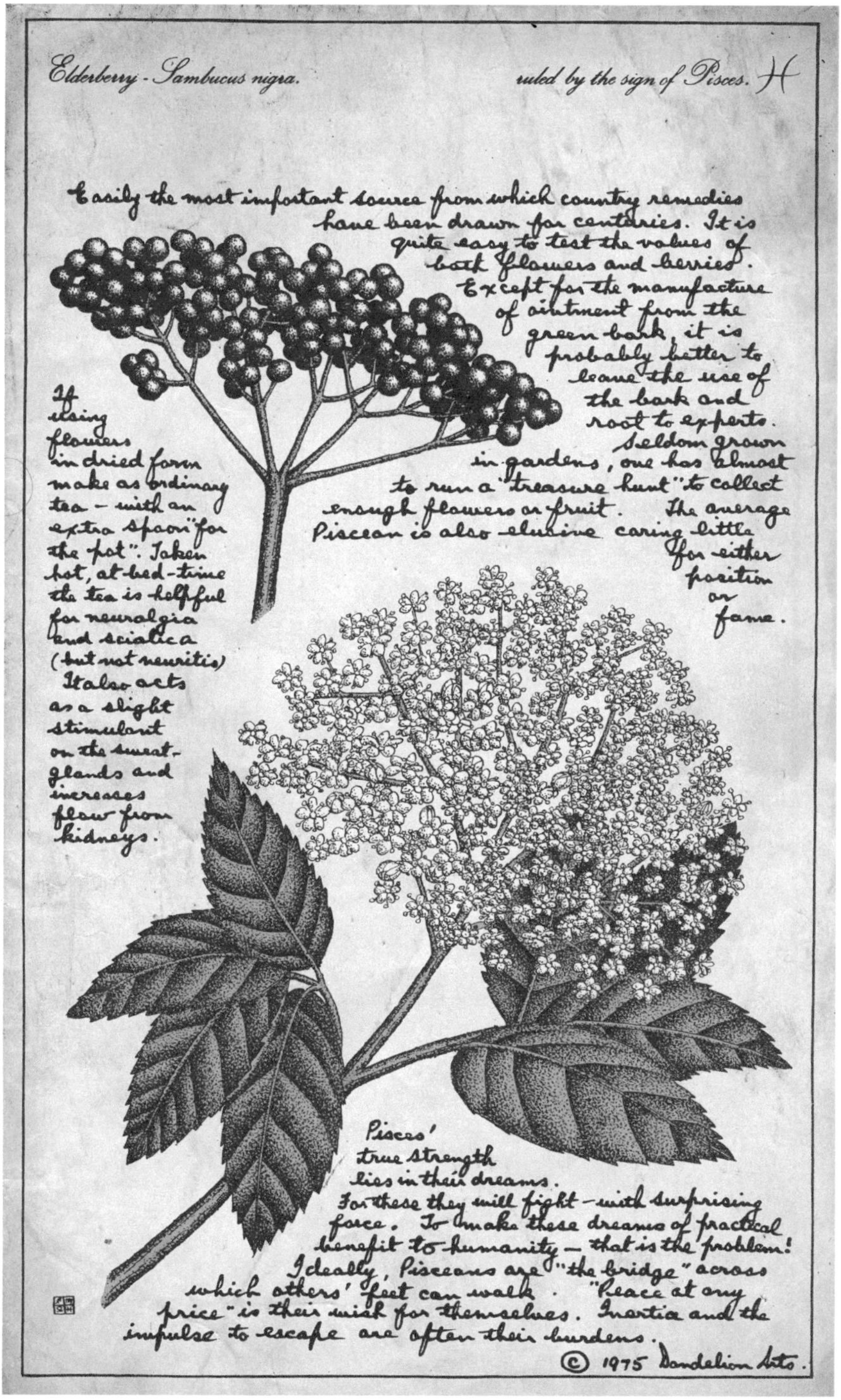
Elderberry - Sambucus nigra.
ruled by the sign of Pisces. ♓
Easily the most important source from which country remedies have been drawn for centuries. It is quite easy to test the values of both flowers and berries. Except for the manufacture of ointment from the green bark, it is probably better to leave the use of the bark and root to experts. Seldom grown in gardens, one has almost to run a "treasure hunt" to collect enough flowers or fruit. The average Piscean is also elusive caring little for either position or fame.
If using flowers in dried form make as ordinary tea – with an extra "spoon for the pot". Taken hot, at bed-time the tea is helpful for neuralgia and sciatica (but not neuritis) It also acts as a slight stimulant on the sweat-glands and increases flow from kidneys.
Pisces' true strength lies in their dreams. For these they will fight – with surprising force. To make these dreams of practical benefit to humanity – that is the problem! Ideally, Pisceans are "the bridge" across which others' feet can walk. "Peace at any price" is their wish for themselves. Inertia and the impulse to escape are often their burdens.
© 1975 Dandelion Arts.

***Note: No one person is 100% representative of their** Zodiac Sign. Most people will know their personal 'Sun Sign' – i.e. the part of the Zodiac the Sun is in at their moment of birth. However, fewer people realize that the 'Moon Sign' and 'Rising Sign' (the Sign of the Zodiac that is located over the eastern horizon at their moment of birth) - plus the Zodiac locations of Mercury, Venus, Mars, etc. - can have a huge impact on a person's way of being too....* ...

That said, Pisces types have deep *soul yearnings* for some form of *escape* from the world. Their spirit motivates them to be wholly *caring*, *compassionate* and *giving* to others on the one hand, while being often *confused*, *vulnerable* and *unfocused* on the other. The Pisces instinct embraces a real need to *transcend* the material existence and find real peace in some *other worldliness*. However, the more negative impulses of Pisces can often lead them to surrender too much fascination for an *unwise cause* or an *overly idealized* loved one. ....
.

As part of this 'Elderberry' herb card indicates... ***"Seldom grown in gardens, one has almost to run a 'treasure hunt' to collect enough flowers or fruit. The average Piscean is also elusive, caring little for either position or fame."...*** ....

HIPPYDIPPYGURU

In ancient Greece, the words "**Know Thyself**" were inscribed over the entrance to the temple of Apollo at Delphi. Visitors to the temple would enter, hoping to discover more about their lives and what they needed to do to ensure better outcomes for themselves. Today, self-knowledge is still as valuable to us now as it ever was - although today we don't need a temple, or a priest, or an oracle, to understand ourselves and our lives better.

The world can be a scary place for us all. Turmoil, conflict and injustice prevail and there seems very little we can do to change it. Yet, as powerless we feel in being able to change our world, we can at least change the one thing that actually affects us and our lives, more than anything else - **ourselves**! And the really interesting thing about this, is that the more we change ourselves, the more the world around us changes too! It may be hard to believe, yet if we make an effort to do it, it will be proven to ourselves over and over again.

HIPPYDIPPYGURU books offer valuable knowledge - knowledge that can help us regain control of ourselves and of our lives. Higher knowledge, focusing on great truths relating to our **Body**, our **Mind**, our **Soul** and our **Spirit**, can enable enormously transformative changes to occur, in terms of our self-understanding in the face of everything behind everything. We welcome you to the brave new world that awaits you!

DISCLAIMER

No information contained within this book - including but not limited to, text, graphics, images or any other material - should be considered as medical advice. The purpose of the 'Healing Herbs of the Zodiac' is to share art that was inspired by traditional astrological and herb-based healing philosophy. It is in no way intended to be a substitute for professional medical advice, diagnosis or treatment. Therefore the publishers accept no responsibility for the material found here and strongly recommends that each individual should always consult the advice of their physician or other qualified health care provider before undertaking any new health care regimen, or implementing anything to be found in this 'Healing Herbs of the Zodiac' publication.